INTERMITTENT FASTING

FOR WOMEN

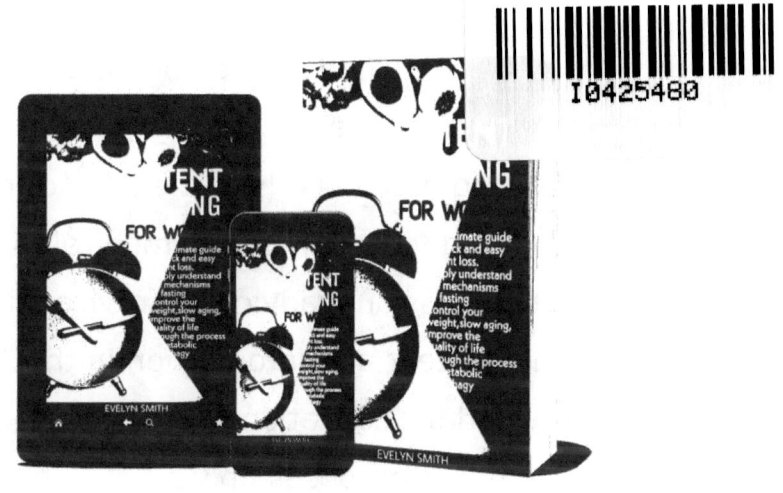

The ultimate guide to quick and easy weight loss.
Simply understand the mechanisms of fasting.
control your weight, slow aging, improve the
quality of life through the process of metabolic
autophagy

Evelyn Smith

Legal & Disclaimer

The information contained in this book and its contents is not designed to replace or take the place of any form of medical or professional advice; and is not meant to replace the need for independent medical, financial, legal or other professional advice or services, as may be required. The content and information in this book has been provided for educational and entertainment purposes only.

The content and information contained in this book has been compiled from sources deemed reliable, and it is accurate to the best of the Author's knowledge, information and belief. However, the Author cannot guarantee its accuracy and validity and cannot be held liable for any errors and/or omissions. Further, changes are periodically made to this book as and when needed.

Where appropriate and/or necessary, you must consult a professional (including but not limited to your doctor, attorney, financial advisor or such other professional advisor) before using any of the suggested remedies, techniques, or information in this book.Upon using the contents and information contained in this book, you agree to hold harmless the Author from and against any damages, costs, and expenses, including any legal fees potentially resulting from the application of any of the information provided by this book. This disclaimer applies to any loss, damages or injury caused by the use and application, whether directly or indirectly, of any advice or information presented, whether for breach of contract, tort, negligence, personal injury, criminal intent, or under any other cause of action.You agree to accept all risks of using the information presented inside this book.You agree that by continuing to read this book, where appropriate and/or necessary, you shall consult a professional (including but not limited to your doctor, attorney, or financial advisor or such other advisor as needed) before using any of the suggested remedies, techniques, or information in this book.

Introduction

A new diet has been introduced for some time: the intermittent fasting diet (also called Intermittent Fasting)

In reality, as we will see better in the course of the article, intermittent fasting is not a real diet but a food program that alternates moments of fasting with intervals on which it is instead allowed to feed.

Intermittent Fasting is becoming increasingly popular as many are the benefits that can be found both physically and psychologically.

Moreover, this type of power supply is also very convenient and practical and adapts very well to our increasingly rapid and frenetic lifestyle.

So if your goal is to lose the extra pounds, then you are in the right place at the right time, because today I will reveal all the details of a truly effective food program proven by various nutritionists.

If you want to learn more then read on below and you will discover the multiple positive effects that you can achieve with the Intermittent Fasting Diet

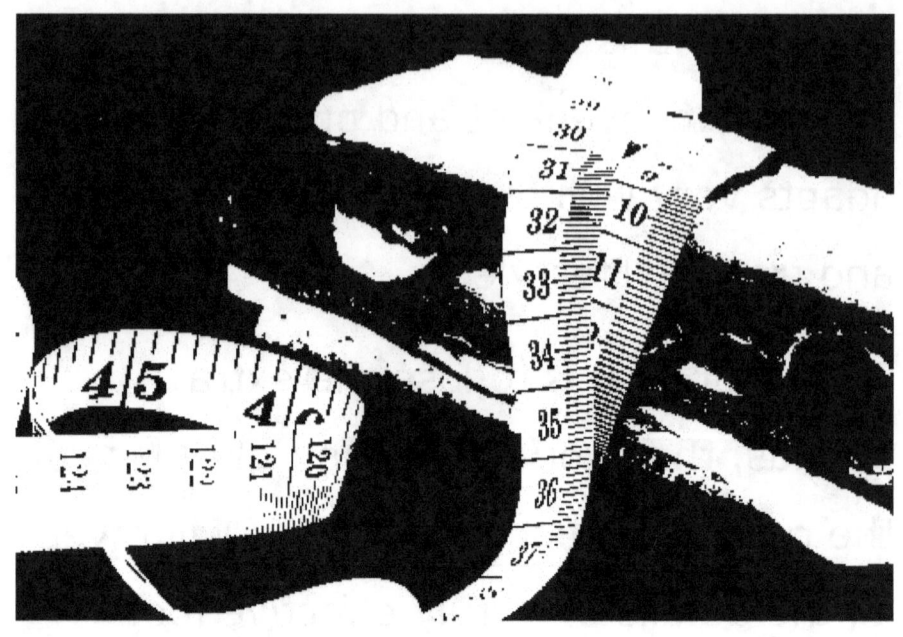

How does intermittent fasting work?

Let's start with the basics ...

What exactly is the diet called "Intermittent Fasting"?

It is a dietary approach in which you will have to enter within the day (or week, depending on the choice you will make when you set the strategic plan), a time of minimum 12-16 hours of fasting, such as to affect the overall caloric balance and hormonal metabolism.

In practice there are two phases:

• a fasting phase called fast, lasting several hours (usually 12 to 20 hours) in which you will not have to introduce any food, except for beverages, such as water, tea, bitter coffee or sugar-free herbal teas

• a phase called fed where you can eat regularly

That's all? That's all.

The Intermittent Fasting is in fact very simple. And that's why it works very well! Soon I'll also explain why.

But first I want to give you some more details.

In fact, there are several methods of intermittent fasting:

1. Intermittent Fasting 16/8: this scheme divides the day into two parts, that is, 8 hours you eat (Fed) and 16 hours of fast (Fast). An example of application is this:

skip breakfast and consume the first meal at noon and then don't eat until 20:00.

2. Every other day (5: 2): for two days a week the calorie intake must be reduced to 500-600 calories, while for the rest of the week you can eat what you want. Of course for this type of diet, the days where the calorie intake is reduced must not be consecutive.

3. Eat stop eat: eat once or twice a week from the evening of the day before until dinner the next day.

As you can see, even in this case they are all extremely simple and allow great flexibility

Intermittent Fasting May Affect Men and Women Differently

There is some evidence that intermittent fasting may not be as beneficial for some women as it is for men.

One study showed that blood sugar control actually worsened in women after three weeks of intermittent fasting, which was not the case in men.

There are also many anecdotal stories of women who have experienced changes to their menstrual cycles after starting intermittent fasting.

Such shifts occur because female bodies are extremely sensitive to calorie restriction.

When calorie intake is low — such as from fasting for too long or too frequently — a small part of the brain called the hypothalamus is affected.

This can disrupt the secretion of gonadotropin-releasing hormone (GnRH), a hormone that helps release two reproductive hormones: luteinizing hormone (LH) and follicle stimulating hormone (FSH).

When these hormones cannot communicate with the ovaries, you run the risk of irregular periods, infertility, poor bone health and other health effects.

Although there are no comparable human studies, tests in rats have shown that 3–6 months of alternate-day fasting caused a reduction in ovary size and irregular reproductive cycles in female rats .

For these reasons, women should consider a modified approach to intermittent fasting, such as shorter fasting periods and fewer fasting days.

Intermittent fasting to lose weight:

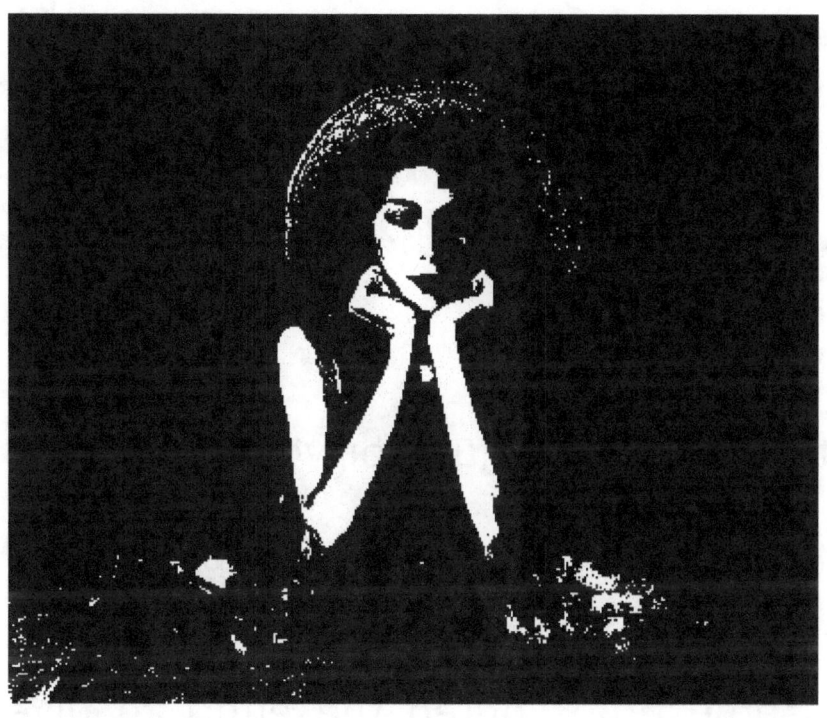

Obviously when we talk about food the first thought goes to the weight and the balance. And therefore to the question: with intermittent fasting is it possible to lose weight?

Absolutely yes! But not only.

If you want to achieve one or all of these three goals:

- Lose weight

- correct various health problems

- live longer

... then this diet is just for you!

In fact it is a great expedient to combine the need to reduce caloric intake and at the same time lighten the effort to give up calories in a natural way.

Having followed many people who wanted to lose weight and who had tried the most varied diets before intermittent fasting, I can say from experience that this methodology is one of those that guarantees the best results.

Not only for the quantity of kilograms lost but above all for the quality of weight loss (very well balanced between lean mass and fat mass) and for ease of weight maintenance once you reach your goal?

How is it possible?

I'll explain why.

There are many people who undertake a diet but very few carry it out. Why do you think? I'll tell you: because it's difficult to give up your favorite foods and because you can't resist the urge to go hungry.

With intermittent fasting, however, both these seemingly insurmountable obstacles are circumvented.

Fasting in fact puts the body in the condition of not having enough energy from food and therefore having to take it from internal reserves (leading to weight loss). Without, however, causing that hunger that we usually feel when we are on a low-calorie diet (reduced in calories).

It seems paradoxical but it is so. Where is the trick?

In the limited duration of fasting.

A prolonged fast in fact demotivates the person, besides putting in place a whole series of compensations from our body, some of which absolutely to be avoided.

While instead fasting only for a limited time makes this practice much easier, because fasting is relatively short and consequently is more bearable.

Other benefits of intermittent fasting

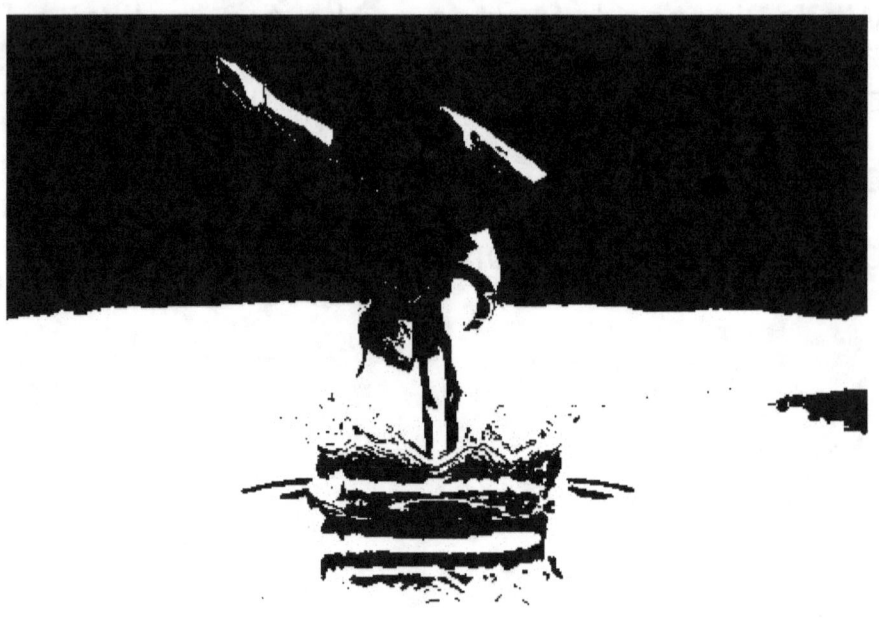

Intermittent Fasting is not only useful for weight loss ... it is a real system to stay healthy for a long time.

In fact, fasting is one of the most powerful means of purifying the body.

When our body is not busy processing food all the time it can devote itself to other activities, such as "cleaning" our body of waste and making many metabolic processes more efficient.

Not to mention the hormonal impact of Intermittent Fasting

Fasting allows us to make our cells more resistant to insulin, promoting protection from important metabolic disorders such as diabetes and the metabolic syndrome.

And finally, during the periods of short fasting, important increases in the production of Growth Hormone have been detected, an important mediator of cell regeneration, useful not only for sportsmen but more generally for all people who wish to slow down the aging process.

How can you guess intermittent fasting is not one of the usual diets that promise miracles in a few weeks.

This is a type of diet that aims to speed up the metabolism and help you lose weight faster by improving cardiovascular health and the immune system in general.

The concept on which it is born is to temporarily disrupt your body and your metabolism, changing the way you usually work your target and forcing it to "wake up" with interesting 360 ° benefits

If you want to undertake this type of diet you will not only lose the extra pounds, but your immune system will become much more resistant to disease.

Many people who have considered this type of diet have felt better physically, and during that time, they felt more energy

Health Benefits of Intermittent Fasting for Women

Intermittent fasting not only benefits your waistline but may also lower your risk of developing a number of chronic diseases.

Heart Health

Heart disease is the leading cause of death worldwide .

High blood pressure, high LDL cholesterol and high triglyceride concentrations are some of the leading risk factors for the development of heart disease.

One study in 16 obese men and women showed intermittent fasting lowered blood pressure by 6% in just eight weeks.

The same study also found that intermittent fasting lowered LDL cholesterol by 25% and triglycerides by 32% .

However, the evidence for the link between intermittent fasting and improved LDL cholesterol and triglyceride levels is not consistent.

A study in 40 normal-weight people found that four weeks of intermittent fasting during the Islamic holiday of Ramadan did not result in a reduction in LDL cholesterol or triglycerides.

Higher-quality studies with more robust methods are needed before researchers can fully understand the effects of intermittent fasting on heart health.

Diabetes

Intermittent fasting may also effectively help manage and reduce your risk of developing diabetes.

Similar to continuous calorie restriction, intermittent fasting appears to reduce some of the risk factors for diabetes.

It does so mainly by lowering insulin levels and reducing insulin resistance.

In a randomized controlled study of more than 100 overweight or obese women, six months of intermittent fasting reduced insulin levels by 29% and insulin resistance by 19%. Blood sugar levels remained the same.

What's more, 8–12 weeks of intermittent fasting has been shown to lower insulin levels by 20–31% and blood sugar levels by 3–6% in individuals with pre-diabetes, a condition in which blood sugar levels are elevated but not high enough to diagnose diabetes .

However, intermittent fasting may not be as beneficial for women as it is for men in terms of blood sugar.

A small study found that blood sugar control worsened for women after 22 days of alternate-day fasting, while there was no adverse effect on blood sugar for men .Despite this side effect, the reduction in insulin and insulin resistance would still likely reduce the risk of diabetes, particularly for individuals with pre-diabetes.

Weight Loss

Intermittent fasting can be a simple and effective way to lose weight when done properly, as regular short-term fasts can help you consume fewer calories and shed pounds.

A number of studies suggest that intermittent fasting is as effective as traditional calorie-restricted diets for short-term weight loss .

A 2018 review of studies in overweight adults found intermittent fasting led to an average weight loss of 15 lbs (6.8 kg) over the course of 3–12 months.

Another review showed intermittent fasting reduced body weight by 3–8% in overweight or obese adults over a period of 3–24 weeks. The review also found that participants reduced their waist circumference by 3–7% over the same period .

It should be noted that the long-term effects of intermittent fasting on weight loss for women remain to be seen.

In the short term, intermittent fasting seems to aid in weight loss. However, the amount you lose will likely depend on the number of calories you consume during non-fasting periods and how long you adhere to the lifestyle.

It May Help You Eat Less

Switching to intermittent fasting may naturally help you eat less.

One study found that young men ate 650 fewer calories per day when their food intake was restricted to a four-hour window .

Another study in 24 healthy men and women looked at the effects of a long, 36-hour fast on eating habits. Despite consuming extra calories on the post-fast day, participants dropped their total calorie balance by 1,900 calories, a significant reduction .

Other Health Benefits

A number of human and animal studies suggest that intermittent fasting may also yield other health benefits.

Reduced inflammation: Some studies show that intermittent fasting can reduce key markers of inflammation. Chronic inflammation can lead to weight gain and various health problems .

Improved psychological well-being: One study found that eight weeks of intermittent fasting decreased depression and binge eating behaviors while improving body image in obese adults .

Increased longevity: Intermittent fasting has been shown to extend lifespan in rats and mice by 33–83%. The effects on longevity in humans is yet to be determined .

Preserve muscle mass: Intermittent fasting appears to be more effective at retaining muscle mass compared to continuous calorie restriction. Higher muscle mass helps you burn more calories, even at rest.

Specifically, the health benefits of intermittent fasting for women need to be studied more extensively in well-designed human studies before any conclusions can be drawn .

Frequently Asked Questions

Here are answers to the most common questions about intermittent fasting.

1. Can I Drink Liquids During the Fast?

Yes. Water, coffee, tea and other non-caloric beverages are fine. Do not add sugar to your coffee. Small amounts of milk or cream may be okay.

Coffee can be particularly beneficial during a fast, as it can blunt hunger.

2. Isn't It Unhealthy to Skip Breakfast?

No. The problem is that most stereotypical breakfast skippers have unhealthy lifestyles. If you make sure to eat healthy food for the rest of the day then the practice is perfectly healthy.

3. Can I Take Supplements While Fasting?

Yes. However, keep in mind that some supplements like fat-soluble vitamins may work better when taken with meals.

4. Can I Work out While Fasted?

Yes, fasted workouts are fine. Some people recommend taking branched-chain amino acids (BCAAs) before a fasted workout.

You can find many BCAA products on Amazon.

5. Will Fasting Cause Muscle Loss?

All weight loss methods can cause muscle loss, which is why it's important to lift weights and keep your protein intake high. One study showed that intermittent fasting causes less muscle loss than regular calorie restriction (16Trusted Source).

6. Will Fasting Slow Down My Metabolism?

No. Studies show that short-term fasts actually boost metabolism (14Trusted Source, 15Trusted Source). However, longer fasts of 3 or more days can suppress metabolism (36Trusted Source).

7. Should Kids Fast?

Allowing your child to fast is probably a bad idea.

Does intermittent fasting work?

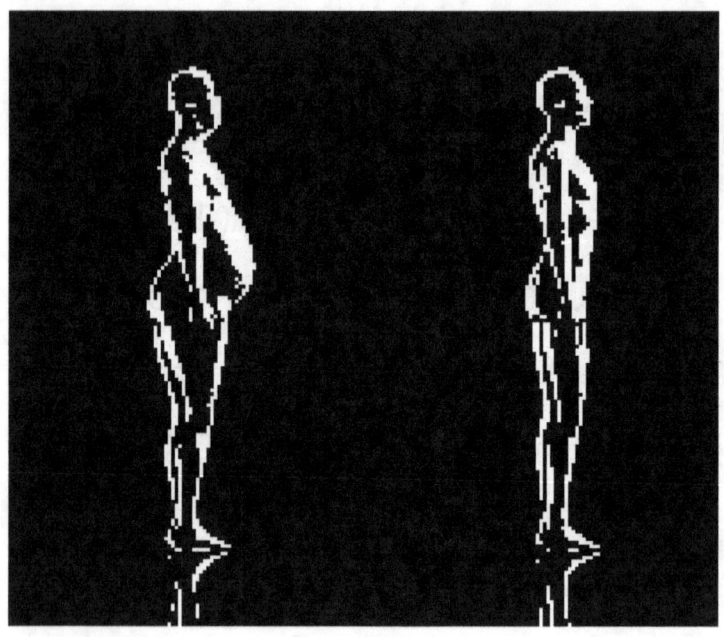

We hear about fasting since ancient times. Many peoples of the world have practiced fasting for purifying, healthy and religious reasons.

And in fact the origins of fasting are lost in the mists of time.

Many even claim that fasting is the "normal mode of functioning of the human being". In fact, if you think about it, over the millennia there has never been such availability of food as it is today.

Therefore the man of the past, for hundreds of thousands of years, has always fasted.

He almost always fasted, at least until the hunters of the tribe could not hunt some big animal, thus giving the possibility to all the various families to take refreshment and "fill up with food"

This phenomenon has happened for a very long time. It is practically inherent in our DNA.

In a world characterized by scarcity of food, the interval of fasting periods more or less long and periods of "binge eating" is practically normal.

This is exactly why intermittent fasting works.

In fact, with the intermittent fasting diet, you introduce nutrients in a cyclic way (the two phases that alternate) and this is a good thing since this regime respects the physiology of the human body.

So, when asked, intermittent fasting works, the answer is certainly yes.

This is a powerful tool that, once you understand how it works, will help you lose excess weight, maintain a healthy weight, live longer and get rid of many diseases.

Types of Intermittent Fasting

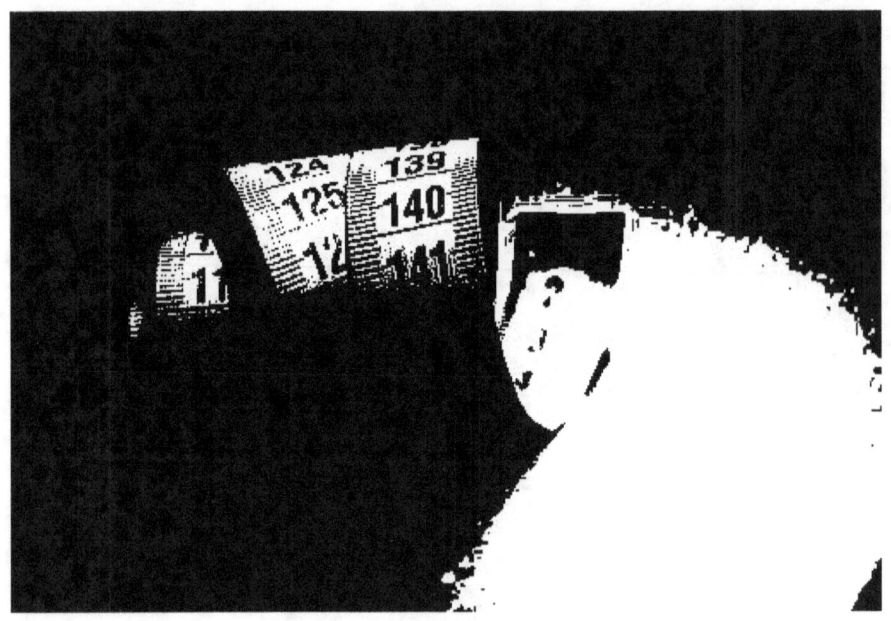

The following are the most popular examples of intermittent fasting and can be adapted as needed. In the Intermittent Fasting Guide you will find an in-depth look at each of the types of fasting listed, which can be associated with a sport.

Diet LeanGains or Intermittent Fasting 16: 8

The LeanGains diet or intermittent fasting 16: 8 provides a feeding window - feeding window - of 8 hours followed by 16 hours of fasting. In the most basic version, we essentially skip breakfast.

Intermittent Fasting 18: 6

Similar to the LeanGains diet. Here the feeding window is 6 hours and fasting for 8 hours.

Fast or 5: 2 diet

For 5 days a week we eat in a classic way. In the remaining two, around 500 calories are consumed.

Warrior Diet or Warrior Diet

The feeding window is 4 hours, usually for dinner. In the rest of the day you can choose to consume fresh vegetables and light fruit.

Alternating Fasting or Alternating-day Fasting

A day of fasting alternates with a day when food is consumed. The day you eat you can choose to do it all day or in a specific feeding window.

OMAD diet

The OMAD diet - One Meal A Day - includes a feeding window of 1 hour a day and 23 hours of fasting. In practice, a full meal a day.

Complete fasting

Once a week or when you want to fast for a whole day. On other days you can choose whether to follow intermittent fasting or not. It is also possible to fast more

lunch, as for example for 5 days.

Best Types of Intermittent Fasting for Women

When it comes to dieting, there is no one-size-fits-all approach. This also applies to intermittent fasting.

Generally speaking, women should take a more relaxed approach to fasting than men.

This may include shorter fasting periods, fewer fasting days and/or consuming a small number of calories on the fasting days.

Here are some of the best types of intermittent fasting for women

Crescendo Method: Fasting 12–16 hours for two to three days a week. Fasting days should be nonconsecutive and spaced evenly across the week (for example, Monday, Wednesday and Friday).

Eat-stop-eat (also called the 24-hour protocol): A 24-hour full fast once or twice a week (maximum of two times a week for women). Start with 14–16 hour fasts and gradually build up.

The 5:2 Diet (also called "The Fast Diet"): Restrict calories to 25% of your usual intake (about 500 calories) for two days a week and eat "normally" the other five days. Allow one day between fasting days.

Modified Alternate-Day Fasting: Fasting every other day but eating "normally" on non-fasting days. You are allowed to consume 20–25% of your usual calorie intake (about 500 calories) on a fasting day.

The 16/8 Method (also called the "Leangains method"): Fasting for 16 hours a day and eating all calories within an eight-hour window. Women are advised to start with 14-hour fasts and eventually build up to 16 hours.

Whichever you choose, it is still important to eat well during the non-fasting periods. If you eat a large amount of unhealthy, calorie-dense foods during the non-fasting periods, you may not experience the same weight loss and health benefits.

At the end of the day, the best approach is one that you can tolerate and sustain in the long-term, and which does not result in any negative health consequences.

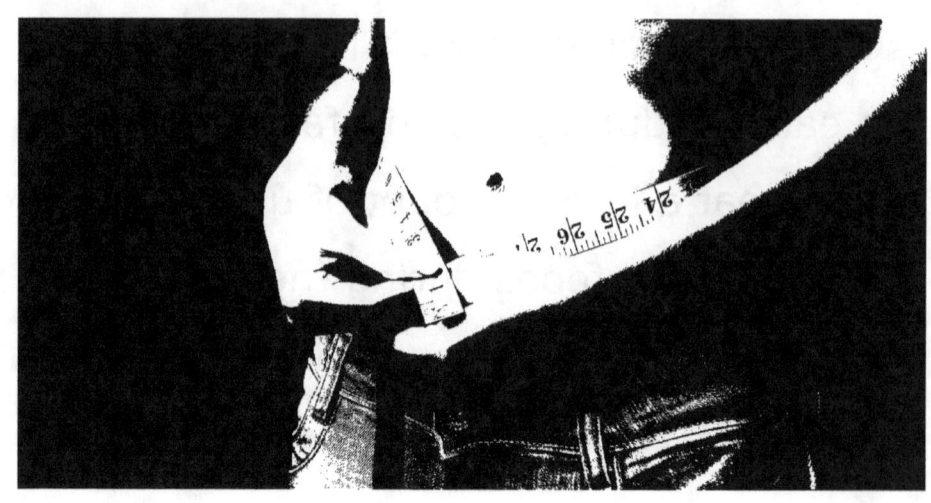

Easier fasting

Yes, because in reality very few people are endowed with the momentum and willpower needed to face a fast that can last up to several days.

Hence the desire for a simpler and more feasible alternative ...

Fasting is one of the most powerful means of resetting unbalanced biochemistry and optimizing conditions that can lead to life extension. But for many people it is difficult to implement, especially for two reasons ...

How is intermittent fasting easier?

Two of the main reasons why prolonged fasting is difficult to implement are the following.

First of all it would be appropriate to take the time dedicated to a prolonged depurative ritual. Then it is advised to set up also the best conditions to operate a fast (to be followed by a nutritionist or by the doctor, to be able to remain focused on this goal, etc.) given the effort required to complete it (it is useless to deny it).

In short, putting a prolonged fasting into practice decidedly difficult makes it difficult if not impossible for many people to approach this healthy practice.

At most, many well-intentioned people simply read something about fasting, try, then get upset and give up and don't try anymore ...

But thanks to intermittent fasting the practice of abstaining from food (and calories in general) becomes decidedly easier for everyone to implement.

Also because unlike prolonged fasting, which may require an interruption of the most demanding activities, intermittent fasting takes advantage of daily tasks

Distract yourself and fast

In what sense does it "take advantage of daily commitments"? pulling a single day without eating can be even easier to bear if you are immersed in your usual activities in the meantime.

So with intermittent fasting there is no need to change anything of one's daily activity rituals. Indeed these can just distract the mind from the thought of food.

A brief workout such as functional training or 30-45 minute yoga on the day of this short fast would even be recommended.

Finally, with a minimum of good will, anyone can FAST and gain health and fitness without necessarily having the mental strength of a fakir.

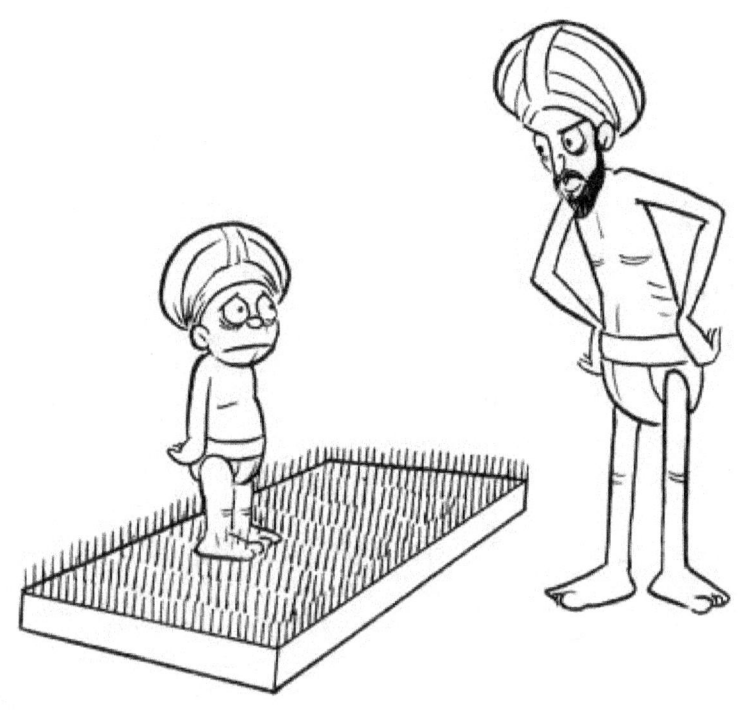

Another grandiose element of intermittent fasting that facilitates its implementation concerns the fact that it is relatively elastic in its duration. That is, the time to devote to fasting is relatively short, therefore bearable

Characteristics of intermittent fasting

Intermittent fasting is an extremely natural way of eating.

During its evolution, the complex and refined metabolism of the human being was forged by an innumerable series of intermittent fasts, not binge eating!

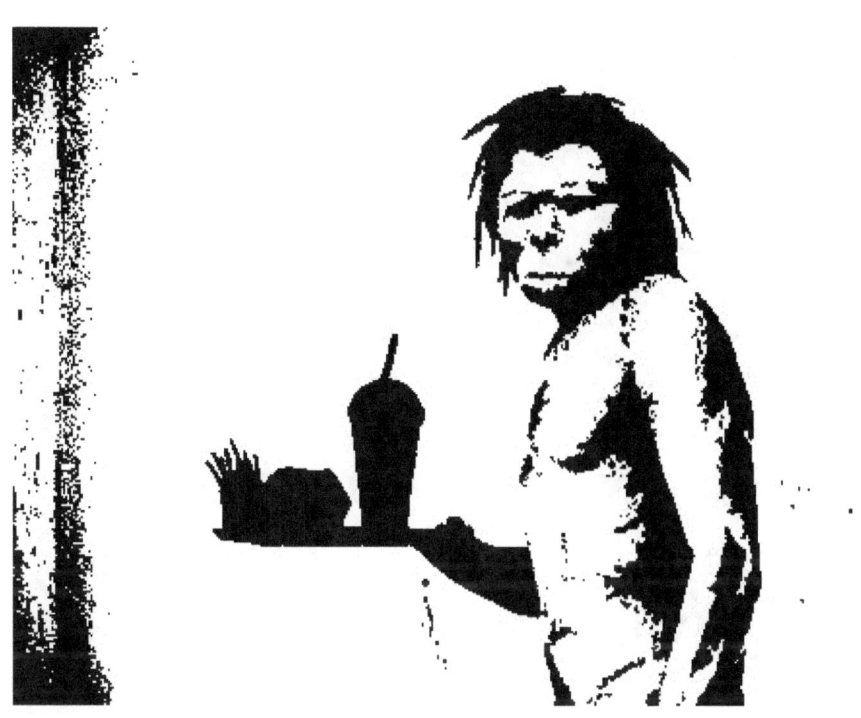

If you think about the difficulty of getting nourishment in nature you can guess that the body has all the means to survive days and days with little or nothing.

Our body is perfectly designed to pass through more or less long periods of absence of food. Not only can it do but it is also a prerogative for its optimal functioning.

It is more normal for us to fast intermittently than to eat 3 or 4 times a day. That is to say, the unhealthy deviation consists precisely in feeding too much, so the remedy is to return to the natural rhythms of intermittent fasting.

Religious fasting

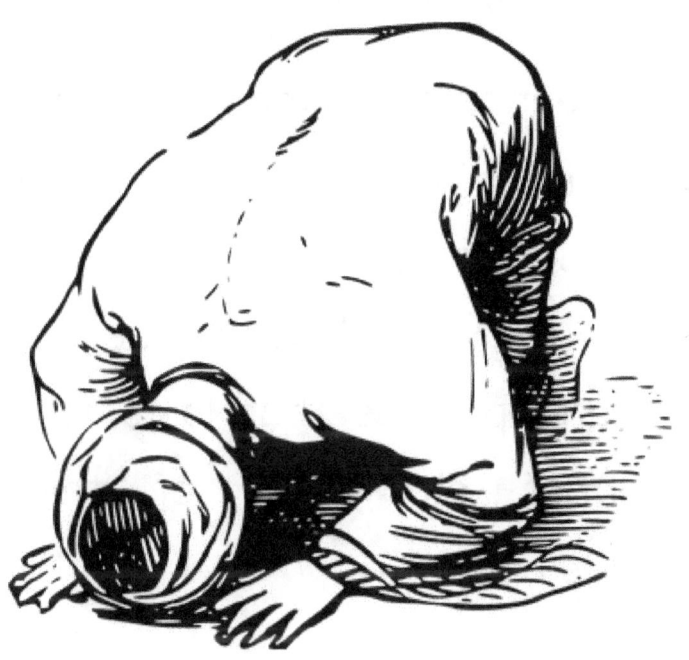

Furthermore, in the course of our most recent evolution, intermittent fasting has continued to be present and widespread for religious reasons. In many different religions and rituals around the world the need has always been felt to devote periods of time to abstaining from food.

Voluntary abstention from food is a form of self-discipline that increases the perception of control that our mind can have on the body. Unleashed desires often cause unhappiness that lasts long after the brief enjoyment of their immediate satisfaction

Fasting = more happiness? maybe yes ..

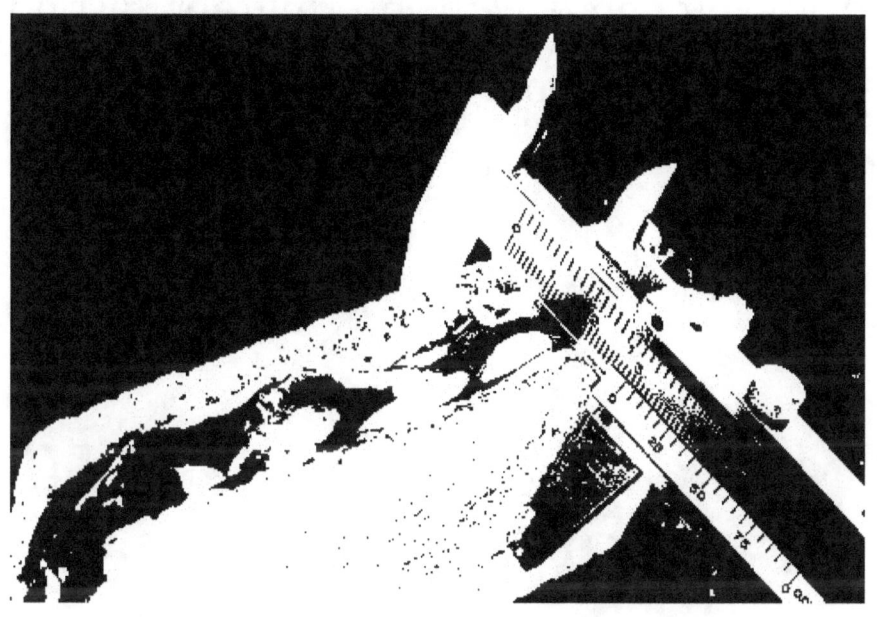

A certain inner solidity due to the fact of "taking back the bridles" of our behavior is associated with greater happiness. This is probably why religions often prescribe programmed food waivers.

Certainly today numerous researches confirm that the metabolic rest that can be implemented with intermittent fasting is one of the most effective and easy to implement ways to get better and live longer

4 ways in which intermittent fasting changes metabolism.

When you stop taking calories for enough time in your body, certain cellular and molecular changes occur ...

1) Activation of autophagy

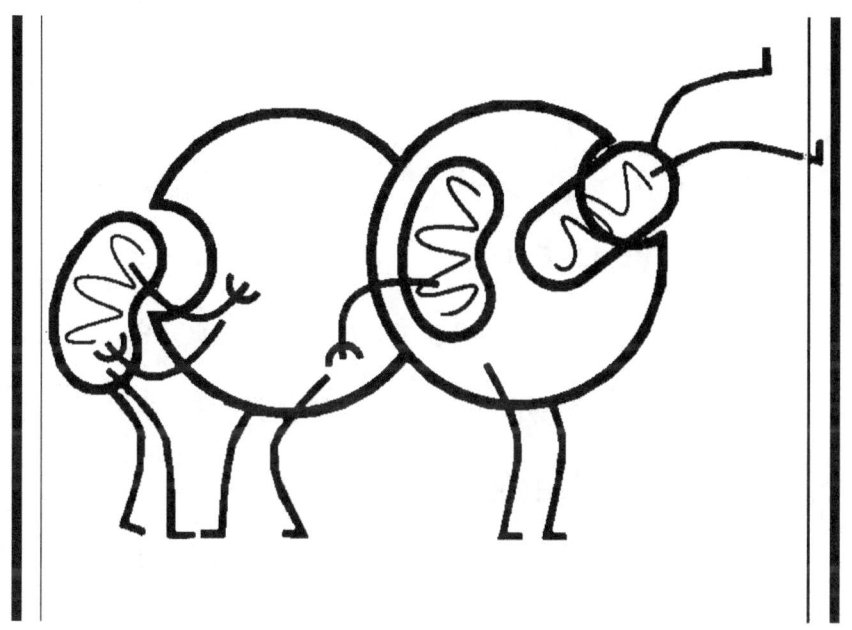

One of the most important events taking

place in a fasting organism is

autophagy1,2. The intelligence of the

body under the stimulus of lack of energy from food sources (during fasting) begins to exploit damaged cells and molecules to feed themselves.

The body thus begins to sustain itself thanks to the use of some of its components now aged and therefore to be replaced. Autophagy in this way expresses two benefits in one: it supplies new energy to the body and at the same time eliminates certain parts that are now dysfunctional.

... AND CELL REGENERATION

Following the elimination of damaged components the body is induced to synthesize new ones. The newly generated components (cells, proteins, etc.) will be healthier than the previous ones because they are just "churned out" by the body's biosynthetic system.

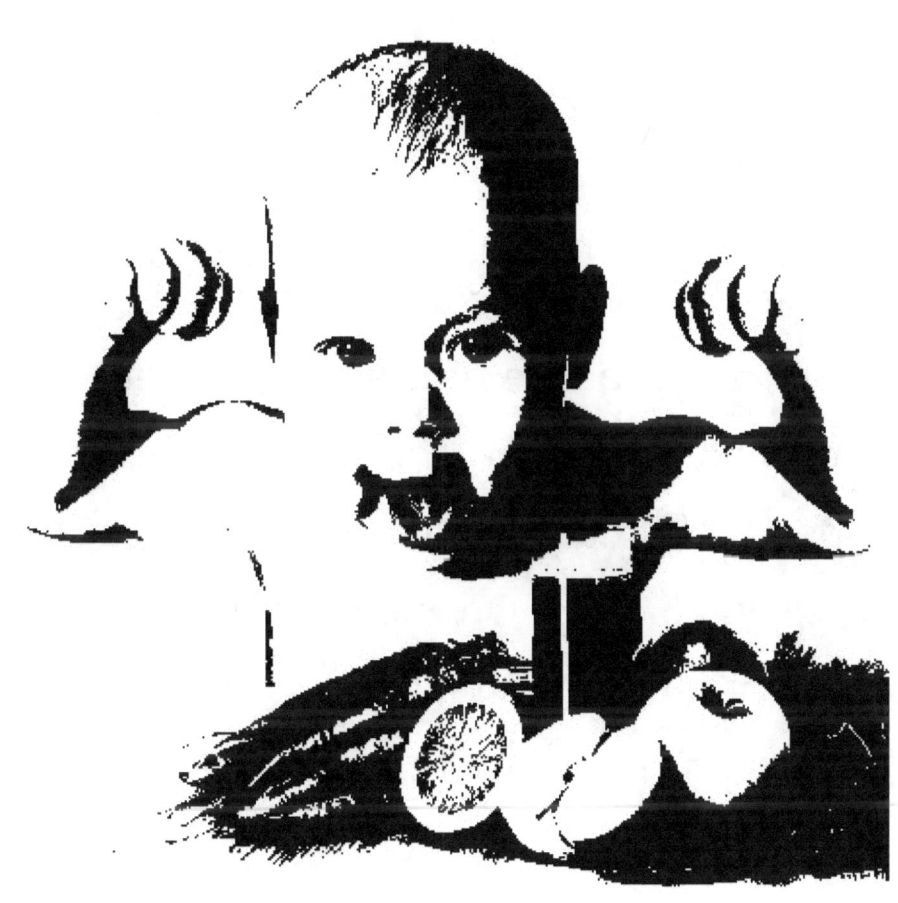

Whenever this cycle of elimination and regeneration occurs, the body is partly renewed and renewed, prolonging its longevity potential.

Not bad...

With a simple short (intermittent) fast the body renews itself.

We had already encountered this process in the practice of the fasting diet. Certainly, however, this last approach is definitely more challenging because it lasts 5 days. On the contrary, an intermittent fasting lasts only from 16 to 24 hours (including the hours of natural night fasting).

2) Synthesis of the GH hormone

GH is the acronym of Growth Hormone, that is growth hormone.

This hormone simultaneously activates the development of muscle mass and the loss of body fat3. Two important benefits for maintaining a lean and healthy body.

The body tends to produce less GH over the years during the aging process. Fasting makes it possible to give a new boost to the production of this important hormone4,5 in a completely natural way

With intermittent fasting the insulin sensitivity improves and consequently the average insulin levels are lowered. This allows easier access to the use of deposited fat reserves

3) Insulin profile

During an intermittent fasting practice several protective action genes are activated. In particular, protective genes are activated against different pathologies7 and genes closely involved in the mechanisms of longevity

The 5 Benefits of Intermittent Fasting # 1) Weight Loss

Intermittent fasting is truly a powerful way to reduce excess fat. Its action on specific hormones such as GH, insulin and noradrenaline makes it an effective tool to reduce abdominal inflammatory fat (see article on belly fat).

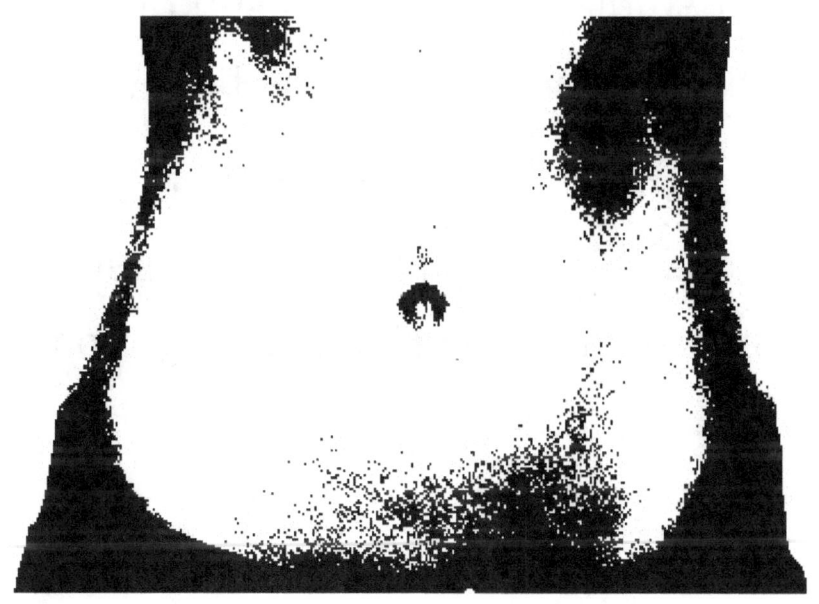

Moreover, even the calorie reduction in the strict sense that occurs during intermittent fasting contributes to weight

2) Anti-inflammatory effect

Several studies show that fasting reduces the inflammatory state of the body9,10.

This leads to a consequent benefit against numerous chronic degenerative pathologies that develop starting from a chronic inflammatory condition.

3) Heart health

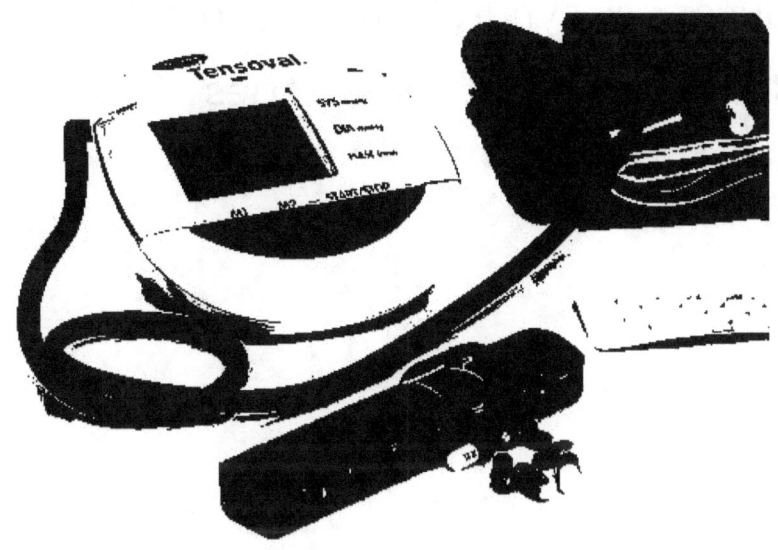

A series of benefits of intermittent fasting linked to heart health 11 makes it particularly suitable for maintaining the cardiovascular system in perfect condition.

Specifically, intermittent fasting can reduce inflammation, blood sugars (improve insulin sensitivity), triglycerides and "bad" LDL cholesterol. All this produces a synergy that promotes the health of the heart and arteries

#4) Antitumor protection

Several studies show a correlation between intermittent fasting and special protection against cancer cells12,13. By now it is becoming increasingly clear how reducing the quantity and frequency of meals can protect better than any other defense against the development of "mad cells"

#5) Maintenance and optimization of brain and nerve functions

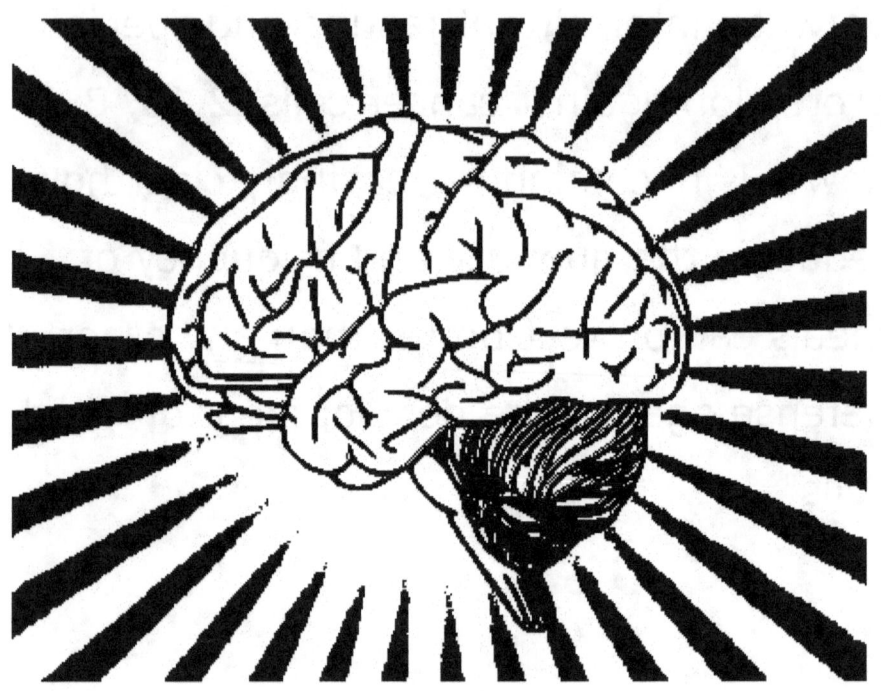

This benefit of intermittent fasting is associated with its general anti-aging effect but is also expressed markedly in relation to neurons.

Some studies show that intermittently fasting stimulates the processes of nerve regeneration15 (postnatal neurogenesis). It also protects against neurodegenerative diseases16.17 and against Alzheimer's disease18.

AND AN ADDITIONAL BENEFIT ...

To this list of 5 points that you have just seen, I would also add another very useful side benefit ... increase your willpower. Willpower is like a muscle that increases its power with training.

More willpower means greater self-control in our lives. A wise and non-violent self-control helps to direct our lives constructively and thus leads us to a greater good

How intermittent fasting works

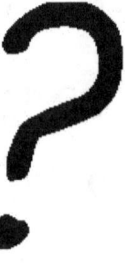

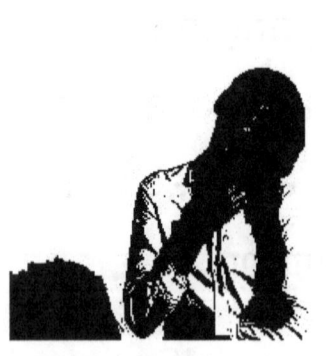

Intermittent fasting is nothing exotic ... who knows how many times you have already put it into practice without knowing it.

Maybe because of the haste and the little time available you missed the breakfast arriving until lunchtime without taking calories of any kind. This is a classic example of intermittent "unconscious" fasting.

One of the most beautiful things that make intermittent fasting easy to follow even for the less "aggressive" is that you can take advantage of the hours of sleep. The hours of sleep are counted in the minimum 16 hours of fasting.

To begin the practice of intermittent fasting you can easily dine and then no longer touch food or calories of any kind until lunchtime the next day.

Indeed...

The time range for caloric abstention is from 16 to 24 hours (uninterrupted). A short time, especially if you think that in this count the hours of sleep are already included.

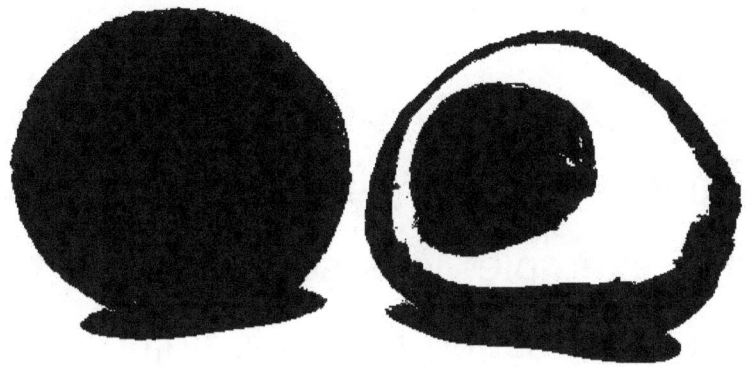

Intermittent fasting easy version

Duration: 16 hours (including overnight fasting).

Mode: starts with dinner, say at 8.00pm. For example, if you finish dinner at 20:30. From that moment on, no food is touched until 12:30 on the following day.

Intermittent fasting Intermediate version

Of course you can decide to make any intermediate version between 16-24 hours. For example, let's say you want to do 18 hours of fasting and finish dinner at 8.30pm ... in this case, don't touch food until 2.30pm the following day.

Intermittent fasting difficult version

Duration: 24 hours (including overnight fasting)

Mode: starts with breakfast for example at 7:00, which you will have finished say at 7:30. Then the intake of calories is interrupted throughout the day and night until breakfast the following day at 7:00.

10 Myths About Fasting and Meal Frequency

Fasting has become increasingly common.

In fact, intermittent fasting, a dietary pattern that cycles between periods of fasting and eating, is often promoted as a miracle diet.

Yet, not everything you've heard about meal frequency and your health is true.

Here are 10 myths about fasting and meal frequency.

1. Skipping breakfast makes you fat

One ongoing myth is that breakfast is the most important meal of the day.

People commonly believe that skipping breakfast leads to excessive hunger, cravings, and weight gain.

One 16-week study in 283 adults with overweight and obesity observed no weight difference between those who ate breakfast and those who didn't .

Thus, breakfast doesn't largely affect your weight, although there may be some individual variability. Some studies even suggest that people who lose weight over the long term tend to eat breakfast .

What's more, children and teenagers who eat breakfast tend to perform better at school .

As such, it's important to pay attention to your specifc needs. Breakfast is beneficial for some people, while others can skip it without any negative consequences.

2. Eating frequently helps reduce hunger

Some people believe that periodic eating helps prevent cravings and excessive hunger.

Yet, the evidence is mixed.

Although some studies suggest that eating more frequent meals leads to reduced hunger, other studies have found no effect or even increased hunger levels .

One study that compared eating three or six high-protein meals per day found that eating three meals reduced hunger more effectively.

That said, responses may depend on the individual. If frequent eating reduces your cravings, it's probably a good idea. Still, there's no evidence that snacking or eating more often reduces hunger for everyone.

3. Eating frequently boosts your metabolism

Many people believe that eating more meals increases your metabolic rate, causing your body to burn more calories overall.

Your body indeed expends some calories digesting meals. This is termed the thermic effect of food TEF.

On average, TEF uses around 10% of your total calorie intake.

However, what matters is the total number of calories you consume — not how many meals you eat.

Eating six 500-calorie meals has the same effect as eating three 1,000-calorie meals. Given an average TEF of 10%, you'll burn 300 calories in both cases.

Numerous studies demonstrate that increasing or decreasing meal frequency does not affect total calories burned

4. Your brain needs a regular supply of dietary glucose

Some people claim that if you don't eat carbs every few hours, your brain will stop functioning.

This is based on the belief that your brain can only use glucose for fuel.

However, your body can easily produce the glucose it needs via a process called gluconeogenesis .

Even during long-term fasting, starvation, or very very-low-carb diets, your body can produce ketone bodies from dietary fats .

Ketone bodies can feed parts of your brain, reducing its glucose requirement significantly.

However, some people report feeling fatigued or shaky when they don't eat for a while. If this applies to you, you should consider keeping snacks on hand or eating more frequently

5. Frequent meals can help you lose weight

Since eating more frequently doesn't boost your metabolism, it likewise doesn't have any effect on weight loss .

Indeed, a study in 16 adults with obesity compared the effects of eating 3 and 6 meals per day and found no difference in weight, fat loss, or appetite .

Some people claim that eating often makes it harder for them to adhere to a healthy diet. However, if you find that eating more often makes it easier for you to eat fewer calories and less junk food, feel free to stick with it.

6. Fasting puts your body in starvation mode

One common argument against intermittent fasting is that it puts your body into starvation mode, thus shutting down your metabolism and preventing you from burning fat.

While it's true that long-term weight loss can reduce the number of calories you burn over time, this happens no matter what weight loss method you use .

There's no evidence that intermittent fasting causes a greater reduction in calories burned than other weight loss strategies.

In fact, short-term fasts may increase your metabolic rate.

This is due to a drastic increase in blood levels of norepinephrine, which stimulates your metabolism and instructs your fat cells to break down body fat.

Studies reveal that fasting for up to 48 hours can boost metabolism by 3.6–14%. However, if you fast much longer, the effects can reverse, decreasing your metabolism.

One study showed that fasting every other day for 22 days did not lead to a reduction in metabolic rate but a 4% loss of fat mass, on average.

7. Your body can only use a certain amount of protein per meal

Some people claim that you can only digest 30 grams of protein per meal and that you should eat every 2–3 hours to maximize muscle gain.

However, this is not supported by science.

Studies show that eating your protein in more frequent doses does not affect muscle mass.

The most important factor for most people is the total amount of protein consumed — not the number of meals it's spread over.

8. Intermittent fasting makes you lose muscle

Some people believe that when you fast, your body starts burning muscle for fuel.

Although this happens with dieting in general, no evidence suggests that it occurs more with intermittent fasting than other methods.

On the other hand, studies indicate that intermittent fasting is better for maintaining muscle mass.

In one review, intermittent fasting caused a similar amount of weight loss as continuous calorie restriction — but with much less reduction in muscle mass .

Another study showed a modest increase in muscle mass for people who consumed all their calories during one huge meal in the evening.

Notably, intermittent fasting is popular among many bodybuilders, who find that it helps maintain muscle alongside a low body fat percentage.

9. Intermittent fasting is bad for your health

While you may have heard rumors that intermittent fasting harms your health, studies reveal that it has several impressive health benefits .

For example, it changes your gene expression related to longevity and immunity and has been shown to prolong lifespan in animals.

It also has major benefits for metabolic health, such as improved insulin sensitivity and reduced oxidative stress, inflammation, and heart disease risk.

It may also boost brain health by elevating levels of brain-derived neurotrophic factor (BDNF), a hormone that may protect against depression and various other mental conditions

10. Intermittent fasting makes you overeat

Some individuals claim that intermittent fasting causes you to overeat during the eating periods.

While it's true that you may compensate for calories lost during a fast by automatically eating a little more afterward, this compensation isn't complete.

One study showed that people who fasted for 24 hours only ended up eating about 500 extra calories the next day — far fewer than the 2,400 calories they'd missed during the fat.Because it reduces overall food intake and insulin levels while boosting metabolism, norepinephrine levels, and human growth hormone (HGH) levels, intermittent fasting makes you lose fat — not gain it.According to one review, fasting for 3–24 weeks caused average weight and belly fat losses of 3–8% and 4–7%, respectively.

As such, intermittent fasting may be one of the most powerful tools to lose weight

What you can drink during intermittent fasting

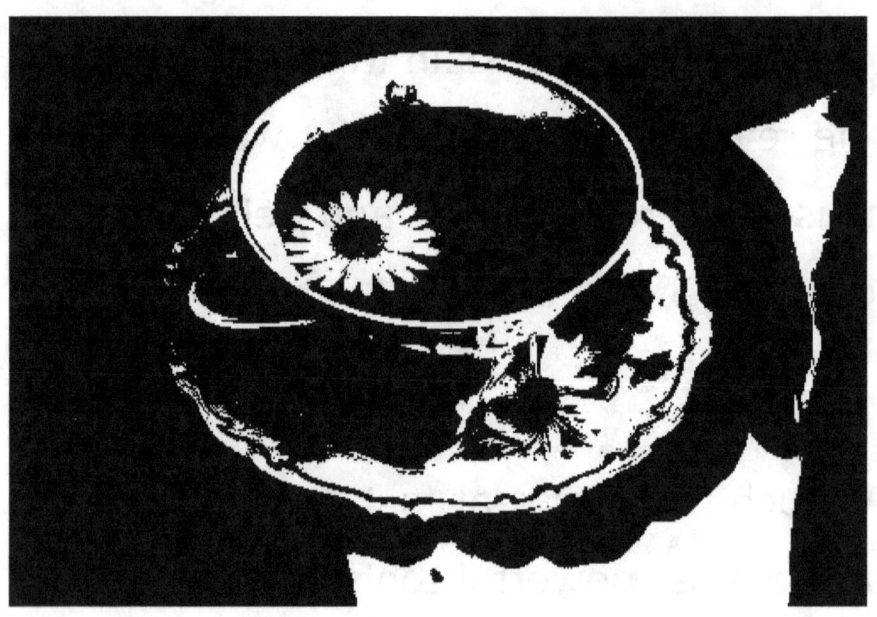

You can drink it at will, indeed it is advisable. Also because good hydration accelerates the metabolism and reduces the sense of hunger. But not all drinks are good for this type of fasting.

The allowed drinks are (without sugar or sweeteners):

Water (possibly in a glass bottle or filtered with an active carbon filter)

Herbal tea (with water not from the tap)

Coffee

You

However, herbal teas, coffee and tea should not be sweetened with sweeteners containing sugar. If you can't do without it you can use some stevia to sweeten without calories and naturally.

The 6 Best Teas to Lose Weight and Belly Fat

Tea is a beverage enjoyed around the world.

You can make it by pouring hot water onto tea leaves and allowing them to steep for several minutes so their flavor infuses into the water.

This aromatic beverage is most commonly made from the leaves of Camellia sinensis, a type of evergreen shrub native to Asia.

Drinking tea has been associated with many health benefits, including protecting cells from damage and reducing the risk of heart disease

Some studies have even found that tea may enhance weight loss and help fight belly fat. Certain types have been found to be more effective than others at achieving this.

Below are six of the best teas for increasing weight loss and decreasing body fat.

1. Green Tea

Green tea is one of the most well-known types of tea, and is linked with many health benefits.

It's also one of the most effective teas for weight loss. There is substantial evidence linking green tea to decreases in both weight and body fat.

In one 2008 study, 60 obese people followed a standardized diet for 12 weeks while regularly drinking either green tea or a placebo.

Over the course of the study, those who drank green tea lost 7.3 pounds (3.3 kg) more weight than the placebo group .

Another study found that people who consumed green tea extract for 12 weeks experienced significant decreases in body weight, body fat and waist circumference, compared to a control group .

This may be because green tea extract is especially high in catechins, naturally occurring antioxidants that may boost your metabolism and increase fat burning .

This same effect also applies to matcha, a highly concentrated type of powdered green tea that contains the same beneficial ingredients as regular green tea.

2. Puerh Tea

Also known as pu'er or pu-erh tea, puerh tea is a type of Chinese black tea that has been fermented.

It is often enjoyed after a meal, and has an earthy aroma that tends to develop the longer it's stored.

Some animal studies have shown that puerh tea may lower blood sugar and blood triglycerides. And studies in animals and humans have shown that puerh tea may be able to help enhance weight loss.

In one study, 70 men were given either a capsule of puerh tea extract or a placebo. After three months, those taking the puerh tea capsule lost approximately 2.2 pounds (1 kg) more than the placebo group.

Another study in rats had similar findings, showing that puerh tea extract had an anti-obesity effect and helped suppress weight gain .

Current research is limited to puerh tea extract, so more research is needed to see if the same effects apply to drinking it as a tea.

3. Black Tea

Black tea is a type of tea that has undergone more oxidation than other types, such as green, white or oolong teas.

Oxidation is a chemical reaction that happens when the tea leaves are exposed to the air, resulting in browning that causes the characteristic dark color of black tea.

There are many different types and blends of black tea available, including popular varieties like Earl Grey and English breakfast.

Several studies have found that black tea could be effective when it comes to weight control.

One study of 111 people found that drinking three cups of black tea each day for three months significantly increased weight loss and reduced waist circumference, compared to drinking a caffeine-matched control beverage.

Some theorize that black tea's potential weight loss effects may be because it's high in flavones, a type of plant pigment with antioxidant properties.

A study followed 4,280 adults over 14 years. It found that those with a higher flavone intake from foods and beverages like black tea had a lower body mass index (BMI) than those with a lower flavone intake.

However, this study looks only at the association between BMI and flavone intake. Further research is needed to account for other factors that may be involved.

4. Oolong Tea

Oolong tea is a traditional Chinese tea that has been partially oxidized, putting it somewhere between green tea and black tea in terms of oxidation and color.

It is often described as having a fruity, fragrant aroma and a unique flavor, though these can vary significantly depending on the level of oxidation.

Several studies have shown that oolong tea could help enhance weight loss by improving fat burning and speeding up metabolism.

In one study, 102 overweight or obese people drank oolong tea every day for six weeks, which may have helped reduce both their body weight and body fat. The researchers proposed the tea did this by improving the metabolism of fat in the body .

Another small study gave men either water or tea for a three-day period, measuring their metabolic rates. Compared to water, oolong tea increased energy expenditure by 2.9%, the equivalent of burning an additional 281 calories per day, on average .

While more studies on the effects of oolong tea are needed, these findings show that oolong could be potentially beneficial for weight loss.

5. White Tea

White tea stands out among other types of tea because it is minimally processed and harvested while the tea plant is still young.

White tea has a distinct flavor very different from other types of tea. It tastes subtle, delicate and slightly sweet.

The benefits of white tea are well-studied, and range from improving oral health to killing cancer cells in some test-tube studies.

Though further research is needed, white tea could also help when it comes to losing weight and body fat.

Studies show that white tea and green tea have comparable amounts of catechins, which may help enhance weight loss .

Furthermore, one test-tube study showed that white tea extract increased the breakdown of fat cells while preventing the formation of new ones .

However, keep in mind that this was a test-tube study, so it's unclear how the effects of white tea may apply to humans.

Additional studies are needed to confirm the potential beneficial effects of white tea when it comes to fat loss.

6. Herbal Tea

Herbal teas involve the infusion of herbs, spices and fruits in hot water.

They differ from traditional teas because they do not typically contain caffeine, and are not made from the leaves of Camellia sinensis.

Popular herbal tea varieties include rooibos tea, ginger tea, rosehip tea and hibiscus tea.

Although the ingredients and formulations of herbal teas can vary significantly, some studies have found that herbal teas may help with weight reduction and fat loss.

In one animal study, researchers gave obese rats an herbal tea, and found that it reduced body weight and helped normalize hormone levels.

Rooibos tea is a type of herbal tea that may be especially effective when it comes to fat burning.

One test-tube study showed that rooibos tea increased fat metabolism and helped block the formation of fat cells.

However, further studies in humans are needed to look into the effects of herbal teas like rooibos on weight loss

Though many people drink tea solely for its soothing quality and delicious taste, each cup may also pack many health benefits.

Replacing high-calorie beverages like juice or soda with tea could help reduce overall calorie intake and lead to weight loss.

Some animal and test-tube studies have also shown that certain types of tea may help increase weight loss while blocking fat cell formation. However, studies in humans are needed to investigate this further.

Additionally, many types of tea are especially high in beneficial compounds like flavones and catechins, which could aid in weight loss as well.

Coupled with a healthy diet and regular exercise, a cup or two of tea each day could help you boost weight loss and prevent harmful belly fat

How many times you have to do intermittent fasting

Now that you understand how to implement an intermittent fasting schedule, it raises a question: How often should you fast?

The answer varies from individual to individual. Most individuals implement the above schedules every week or every other week. If you're new to fasting, start with a moderate schedule, trying it every other week or every three weeks. If your body adapts well, aim for a regular, weekly schedule.

There's no wrong answer here. Pay close attention to how your body responds to your fasting schedule, and adjust as needed. Keep in mind that life changes can happen. You may need to tweak your schedule to allow for social gatherings, vacations and physical activity or competition.

In general, once or twice a week is an optimal frequency to perform intermittent fasting.

What not to eat during intermittent fasting

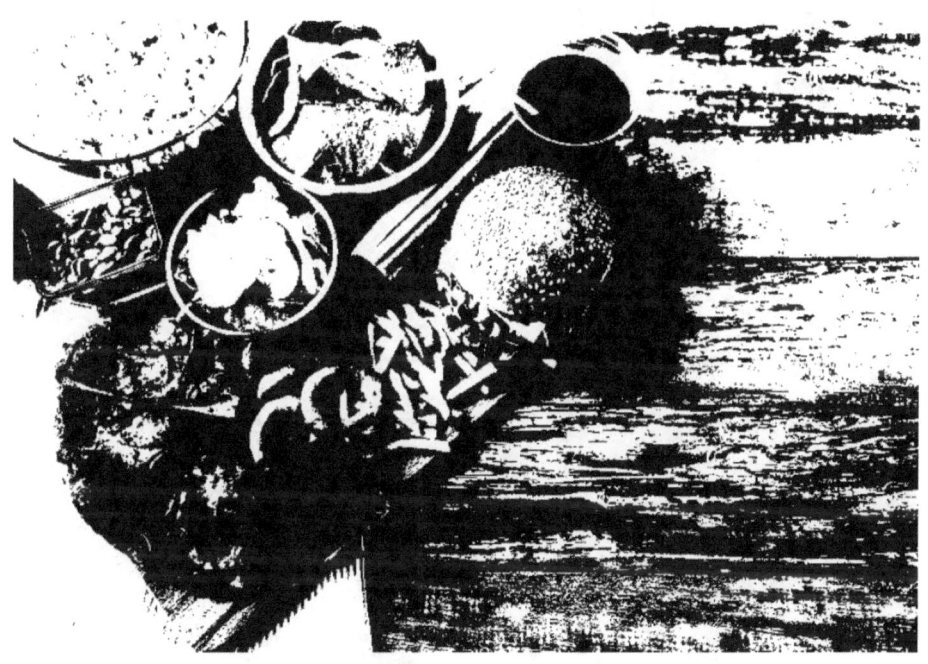

Any source of calories should be avoided during the period of intermittent fasting. So also all the oils and obviously sugars.

Any solid food should be avoided, including fruits, seeds and vegetables. Even shredded versions, extracts and juices are NOT used during the period of intermittent fasting.

Who should not do intermittent fasting

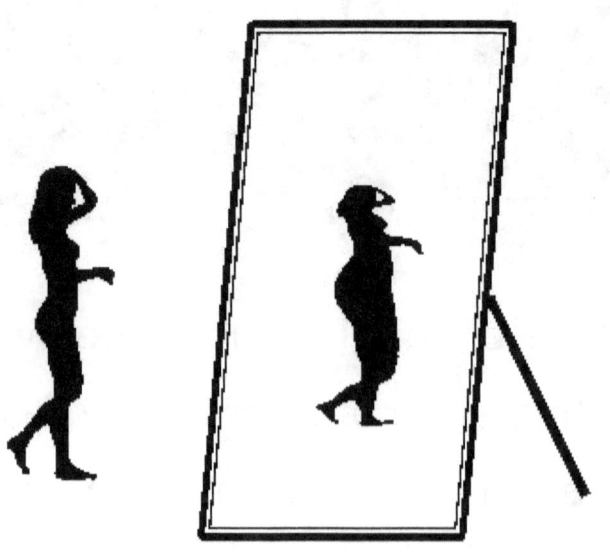

If you suffer or have suffered from eating disorders, it is not recommended to face any type of calorie restriction.

It is not appropriate for children to follow an intermittent fast.

Women in general should address it in the less aggressive version by 16 hours no more than 1-2 times a week. In fact, some women may be affected by hormonal changes (increased testosterone) which could lead to amenorrhea.

If the woman suffers from infertility she should avoid intermittent fasting.

In any case of pre-existing conditions it is necessary to discuss with your doctor to see if in the specific case it is advantageous to deal with the practice of intermittent fasting.

Who can deal with intermittent fasting

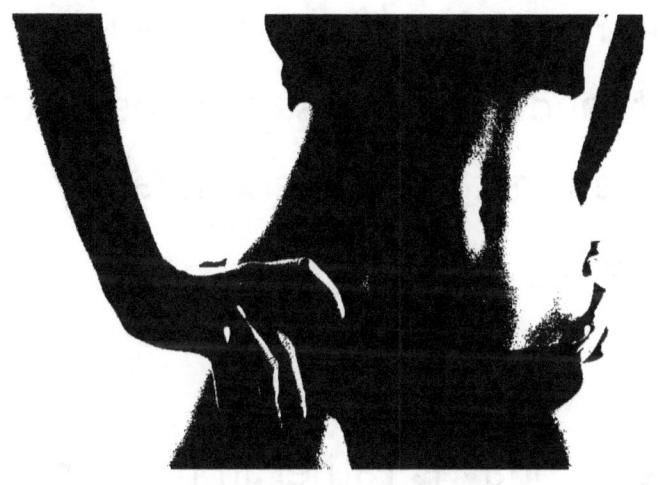

In general, boys are the ones who only benefit from intermittent fasting.

All people (except children) are healthy, especially if overweight can benefit enormously from intermittent fasting.

As indicated in the initial part of the article, the human being in the course of its evolution has always had to confront the lack of food. Eating less and less often is one of the most natural and healthy things there is.

The problem today is rather in the sense of excess. How many diseases are caused by unhealthy foods consumed in excess!

Intermittent fasting is the (simple) turn we need

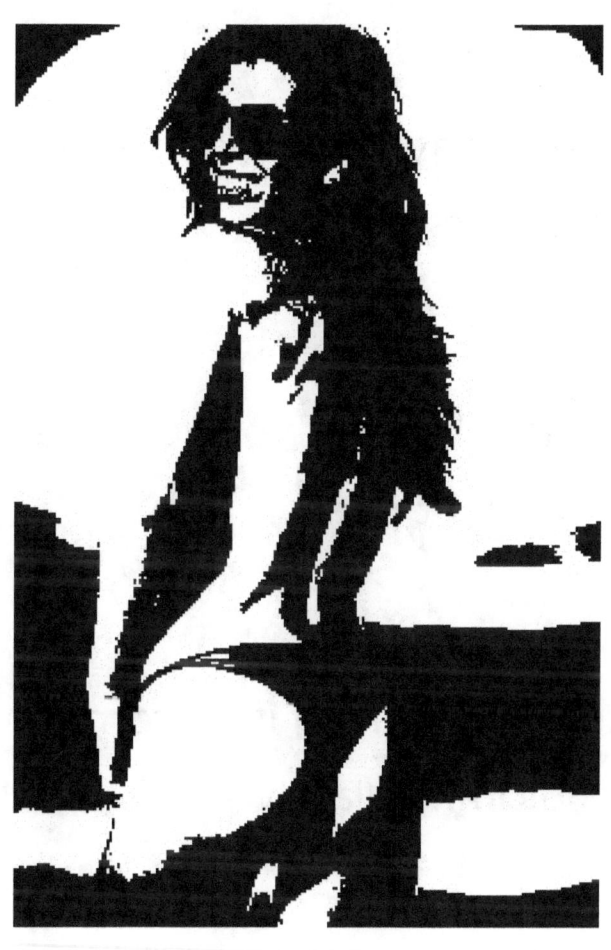

... It is appropriate to correct this trend as soon as possible by turning to the healthy habit of intermittently fasting.

There is a way of saying oriental wisdom that suggests ...

"No matter how far you've gotten away from the right path ... turn!"

The important thing is to correct yourself and do it immediately.

The more you continue in the same (wrong) direction under the influence of inertia, the more you will drift away: turning, now!

Conclusions

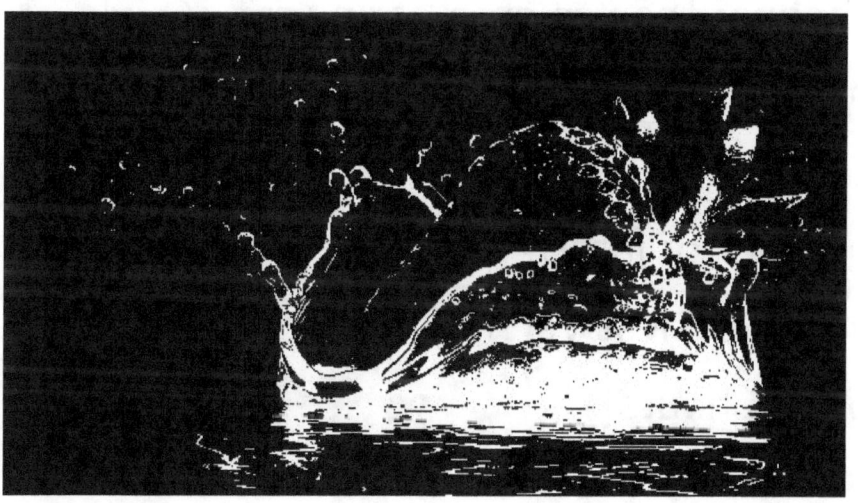

Are you lazy but want to do something more to regain health and fitness?

Intermittent fasting has all the characteristics to unleash a great therapeutic, protective and slimming power.

There is nothing healthier, simpler and cheaper than to stop eating for 16-24 hours 1-2 times a week. You can also count the 7-8 hours of sleep in the total number of intermittent fasting hours (so in the easiest version it is like fasting for only 8 hours!).

On the practical side, fasting intermittently also facilitates life. In fact, skipping a couple of meals every now and then eliminates the need to prepare them and you recover some time to devote to something else.

Motivation: Intermittet fasting success stories

Intermittent Fasting Success Stories

1. lucy's Story

After one year of 4:3 intermittent fasting, I've lost 39.8kg (6 stone 3.8lb). My body mass index (BMI) has reduced by 12.28, down to 36.79 from 49.07. I have had to throw many of my old clothes out because they have become loose and comical.

During the second half of my fasting (the latter six months of the twelve), I experienced long plateau periods, meaning little weight loss was apparent due to my metabolism slowing and my body burning fewer calories, strangely, these plateaus seem to only occur when approaching a weight-loss milestone (130kgs, 120kgs), and were usually followed by an abrupt and substantial loss of weight. Whilst I am aware that plateau is quite common around the six to nine-month mark of dieting, I am hoping to get past it and speed up my weight loss process.

I find it is easy to do after a year. On most fasting days, I often eat nothing at all, and sometimes continue the fasting until my afternoon meal the next day if I am not overly hungry.

All in all, I feel fantastic, although I still carry a lot of body weight, I feel much lighter on my feet and more energetic than I was before. I also feel as though my strength and endurance have improved.

2. Tabatha's Story

I have had to throw all of my old clothes out and purchase an entirely new wardrobe since fasting. I have just turned 65, my weight is now 127lbs, my body-fat ratio is 27.3%, I have a BMI of 20.2%, and a 29-inch waistline. I am feeling very good and am planning on continuing my dietary plan for a few years or more, to ensure I remain healthy and enjoy the years I have left to the fullest.Here's how I achieved it:

I use the 5:2 method, whereby I only had to count calories on two days out of seven in a week.During the early stages of the regime I would nibble on snacks the evening before fast days to load up on calories, and the next day whilst fasting I would be thinking about food non-stop. However, this didn't last that long, and it wasn't long before I stopped snacking even on non-fasting days.

I found that distributing my calorie intake between the times of 12 pm and 7 pm, and skipping breakfast everyday (as I had always struggled to consume and enjoy breakfast consistently) worked wonders for me.

Once I hit my target weight in March, I decided to change to a 6:1 plan to see how my body would react. What I found was that even when I didn't fast at all throughout the week by adhering to the 7-hour window (between 12 pm and 7 pm), I was still steadily losing weight. After reading some intermittent fasting success stories, I found that this seven-hour window had been useful for others, too.

After going on holiday, I put on a few pounds, but once I had returned home and re-established my seven hour eating window, I lost the extra holiday weight within two weeks.

3. Jina's Story

After deciding that it was time to change my eating habits and attain what is considered a healthy weight for my age, I decided to try 5:2 intermittent fasting. I began fasting on the 1st of July 2013, and my body weight was 170lbs (12st 2lbs), as of today (September 24th, 2013), my body weight has dropped to 145lbs (10st 5lbs).

I generally fast on Mondays, Thursdays, or Fridays, depending on impending commitments. I fast from evening meal to evening meal, for 24 hour periods. At one point I attempted to fast for a 36-hour period, but this caused me to have trouble sleeping and left my stomach feeling extremely empty. For this reason, I continued to consume a small, nutritious meal in the evening on fast days.

I began diet by eating complex carbohydrates (whole meal bread, spaghetti, and brown rice), but have swapped these starchy foods for courgette "spaghetti" and cauliflower "rice", which are delicious alternatives. I have abstained from eating all white carbohydrates, and I log everything I eat into an app on my smart phone which records the calorie content. This provides me with helpful statistics and ensures I adhere to my weight loss goals.

Since fasting I have gone from a size 16 to a size 10, and I am feeling very positive about my appearance. I have read many intermittent fasting success stories to ascertain that I am not alone in my success. I will continue to maintain my fasting plan and work toward my target weight of 139lbs (9st 13lbs).

4. Maria's Story

After putting a few stone on during menopause, I decided to try intermittent fasting to lose my post-menopausal weight. Starting in September/October time in 2012, I first implemented the 5:2 diet plan but soon began a 16/8 method, wherein I would have 16 hour fast periods and 8 hour eating windows every day. I get great displeasure from counting calories so I found this method best suited for more – simply skip breakfast and don't nibble in the evenings, how hard could it be? Since fasting I have gone from 140lbs (10st) to around 112/117lbs (8st to 8st 4lbs).

At first I would eat whatever I wanted during the 8 hour eating period of each day, with little to no concern of healthy/nutritious meals. Before long, I began to implement healthier meals and really noticed the benefits from doing so.

At first, weight loss was slow, which can be disheartening, but I persevered and eventually lost the weight I wanted to. I feel brilliant, full of energy and life, and my friends and family say I look better than I have for many years. Intermittent fasting truly has changed my life for the better. I would definitely recommend this method of eating, and this way of life to anyone.

www.ingramcontent.com/pod-product-compliance
Lightning Source LLC
Chambersburg PA
CBHW072134280526
45788CB00002B/631